EMRO Technical Publications Series 39

Atlas: child, adolescent and maternal mental health resources in the Eastern Mediterranean Region

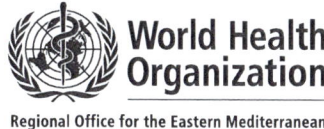

Regional Office for the Eastern Mediterranean

WHO Library Cataloguing in Publication Data

World Health Organization. Regional Office for the Eastern Mediterranean
   Atlas: child, adolescent and maternal mental health resources in the Eastern Mediterranean Region: / World Health Organization. Regional Office for the Eastern Mediterranean
   p. ..- (EMRO Technical Publications Series; 39)
1. Mental Health Services - statistics & numerical data - Eastern Mediterranean Region 2. Adolescent Health Services - statistics & numerical data 3. Child Health Services - statistics & numerical data 4. Health Resources 5. Health Care Surveys - statistics & numerical data I. Title II. Regional Office for the Eastern Mediterranean III. Series
   ISBN: 978-92-9021-796-1   (NLM Classification: WM 16)
   ISBN: 978-92-9021-798-5 (online)
   ISSN : 1020-0428

© World Health Organization 2011
All rights reserved.

The designations employed and the presentation of the material in this publication do not imply the expression of any opinion whatsoever on the part of the World Health Organization concerning the legal status of any country, territory, city or area or of its authorities, or concerning the delimitation of its frontiers or boundaries. Dotted lines on maps represent approximate border lines for which there may not yet be full agreement.

The mention of specific companies or of certain manufacturers' products does not imply that they are endorsed or recommended by the World Health Organization in preference to others of a similar nature that are not mentioned. Errors and omissions excepted, the names of proprietary products are distinguished by initial capital letters.

All reasonable precautions have been taken by the World Health Organization to verify the information contained in this publication. However, the published material is being distributed without warranty of any kind, either expressed or implied. The responsibility for the interpretation and use of the material lies with the reader. In no event shall the World Health Organization be liable for damages arising from its use.

Publications of the World Health Organization can be obtained from Distribution and Sales, World Health Organization, Regional Office for the Eastern Mediterranean, PO Box 7608, Nasr City, Cairo 11371, Egypt (tel: +202 2670 2535, fax: +202 2670 2492; email: PAM@emro.who.int). Requests for permission to reproduce, in part or in whole, or to translate publications of WHO Regional Office for the Eastern Mediterranean – whether for sale or for noncommercial distribution – should be addressed to WHO Regional Office for the Eastern Mediterranean, at the above address: email: WAP@emro.who.int.

Design, layout and printing by WHO Regional Office for the Eastern Mediterranean, Cairo, Egypt

Contents

Preface 5

Acknowledgments 6

1. Introduction 7
1.1 Background 7
1.2 WHO Eastern Mediterranean Region 7
1.3 Atlas projects 8
1.4 Objectives of the Atlas 8
1.5 Methods and limitations 9

2. Public policy and legislation 10
2.1 Child and adolescent mental health 10
2.2 Maternal mental health 10

3. Mental health services 11
3.1 Child and adolescent mental health 11
3.2 Maternal mental health 13

4. Health care financing 16

5. Human resources 16
5.1 Child and adolescent mental health 16
5.2 Maternal mental health 17

6. Data collection and quality assurance 18

7. Medications and other treatment modalities 20

8. Child and adolescent mental health promotion and prevention of psychiatric problems 22

9. Religion and mental health 22

10. Key findings 23

References 25

Annexes 27

Preface

Atlas: child, adolescent and maternal mental health resources in the Eastern Mediterranean Region has been specifically designed to map child, adolescent and maternal mental health resources in countries of the Region. The data collection tool and methodology were modelled on an earlier WHO global exercise conducted in 2005 to map child and adolescent mental health resources. However, in the earlier exercise only eight countries of the Region, comprising 38.5% of the regional population participated. The current publication was developed as part of the activities outlined in the regional strategic directions for child, adolescent and maternal mental health approved by the Regional Committee for the Eastern Mediterranean in its 57th session in 2010. It is distinct from the earlier version in two main respects. First, it focuses exclusively on countries of the Region with their distinct demographic, cultural, religious and social attributes. Second, it maps mental health resources available for maternal mental health, in addition to child and adolescent mental health resources in countries of the Region. The tool assessed a number of key components: 1) public policy and legislation; 2) mental health services; 3) health care financing 4) human resources; 5) data collection and quality assurance; 6) medications and other treatment modalities; 7) promotion and prevention of psychiatric problems; and 8) religion and mental health.

The Atlas was developed based on an assessment conducted in individual countries. Data from individual countries were collected through key focal points in ministries of health using secondary data sources, surveys and aided by a team conducting focus groups and key informant interviews. This report summarizes the information collected for 19 out of the 23 countries of the Region. Data are presented for all eight domains of the tool.

This publication is aimed at policy-makers, health system managers and mental health professionals, as well as lay readers interested in child, adolescent and maternal mental health issues. It will assist countries in identifying the main gaps and weaknesses and developing information-based policies and plans with clear baseline information and targets. Moreover, countries will be able to monitor progress in implementation of policies and legislation, and chart progress in the provision of community-based services. It is hoped that the process of data collection will have stimulated system-level thinking by governments and health system managers and prompt them to build a data infrastructure, implement data system improvements and build a network for mental health action, in general, and for child, adolescent and maternal mental health, in particular. The publication can also serve as a potent advocacy tool for facilitating improvements in mental health services, and over time, for combating the stigma attached to mental health, based on evidence from the Eastern Mediterranean Region.

Acknowledgments

ATLAS – Child, adolescent and maternal mental health resources in the Eastern Mediterranean Region was conceptualized after the 2005 global WHO Atlas project to map child and adolescent mental health resources but with an additional focus on maternal mental health resources. The data collection tool and methodology, modelled on an earlier WHO global exercise conducted in 2005, were further developed through the collaborative efforts of the Mental Health and Substance Abuse programme of the WHO Regional Office for the Eastern Mediterranean and the Harvard Medical School Children's Hospital of Boston Global Partnerships in Psychiatry.

Management of the project at the WHO Regional Office for the Eastern Mediterranean was provided by Dr Haifa Madi, Director, Division of Health Protection and Promotion, and Professor Myron Belfers at the Harvard Medical School Children's Hospital of Boston Global Partnerships in Psychiatry. Dr Hesham Hamoda, Harvard Medical School Children's Hospital of Boston Global Partnerships in Psychiatry, and Dr Khalid Saeed, WHO Regional Office for the Eastern Mediterranean, were actively involved in developing the data collection tools, reviewing country data, providing feedback to country participants, analysing data and drafting this report. Dr Chiara Servili provided additional technical input and feedback.

Collaborators in 19 countries and territories participated in collecting the data for this study in child, adolescent and maternal mental health resources in the Eastern Mediterranean. They are as follows. Afghanistan: Alia Ibrahimzai; Bahrain: Sharifa Bucheeri; Djibouti: Idd Waîs Ibrahim; Egypt: Fahmy Bahgat; Islamic Republic of Iran: A Hadjebii; Iraq: Emad A. Abdulghani; Kuwait: Haya Al-Mutairi; Libyan Arab Jamahiriya: Ali M. Elroey; Morocco: Fatima Asouab, Fadoua Rahhaoui and Soumaya Rachidi; Oman: Mahmoud Al Abri; Pakistan: Fareed Aslam Minhas; Saudi Arabia: Abdulhameed A. Al-Habeeb; Somalia: Abdi Rahman Ali Awale; Sudan: Zeinat Billa Sanhouri; Syrian Arab Republic: Eyad Yanis; Tunisia: Samira Milad; United Arab Emirates: Saleha K. Bin Thiban; Occupied Palestinian territory: Hazem Ashour; Yemen: Mohamed A. Al-Khulaidi.Mr Peter Forbes at the Children's Hospital in Boston provided assistance with the statistical analysis and graphics with the support of the Stuart J. Goldman Award for conducting this work.

1. Introduction

1.1 Background

Mounting evidence suggests that antecedents of adult mental disorders can be traced to childhood and adolescence, and that preventive and curative interventions can reduce the burden of mental health disorders during childhood and later on in life (1–3). Yet, the development of policies and programmes for child and adolescent mental health clearly lag behind those for adult mental health (4). The reasons for this include widespread lack of awareness about child development and childhood mental disorders, relatively weak advocacy, lack of trained human resources and training programmes, and a paucity of reliable data on the epidemiology of child and adolescent psychiatric disorders (5,6). In addition, the lack of systematic mapping of existing child and adolescent mental health services and resources is a significant impediment towards strategic planning and the effective allocation of scarce resources.

Maternal mental health problems pose a significant burden for women, their children, families, and communities at large. Women's mental health requires special considerations in view of the greater likelihood of women suffering from depression and anxiety disorders, as well as the impact of their mental health on childbearing and childrearing (7). Women are also at increased risk of suffering from mental health problems such as postpartum depression and postpartum psychosis following delivery, which can lead to significant morbidity and mortality through suicide or infantile homicide (8). The linkage between maternal mental health and child and adolescent mental health is now so evident that this Atlas includes, and attempts to integrate, both domains.

This publication compiles data on available resources for maternal, child and adolescent mental health in the Eastern Mediterranean Region. These data enable an analysis of current resources and identification of service gaps. Such information is of paramount importance for planning and service development in the Region to provide mental health services for a significant proportion of the population.

1.2 WHO Eastern Mediterranean Region

Up until September 2011, the WHO Eastern Mediterranean Region comprised 22 countries and territories: Afghanistan, Bahrain, Djibouti, Egypt, Islamic Republic of Iran, Iraq, Jordan, Kuwait, Lebanon, Libyan Arab Jamahiriya, Morocco, Oman, Pakistan, occupied Palestinian territory, Qatar, Saudi Arabia, Somalia, Sudan, Syrian Arab Republic, Tunisia, United Arab Emirates and Yemen.[1]

Countries of the Region are undergoing rapid demographic and socioeconomic transition. The demographics of countries in this Region are notable for high fertility and population growth rates and a high percentage of the population is under 18 years of age. In fact, almost half of the population of countries such as Yemen, Somalia, occupied Palestinian territory and Sudan (including south Sudan) is under 15 years of age (9). The Region has also witnessed several wars and humanitarian crises to which women and children are among the most vulnerable. Exposure to these potentially traumatic events can lead to long-term consequences. Such demographic and sociopolitical characteristics underscore the importance of understanding mental health

---

[1] The country assessments that inform this report were conducted in 2010, before South Sudan became an independent Member State in the Region in September 2011. Thus, the information contained in the report does not provide disaggregated data for Sudan and South Sudan.

needs and subsequently providing mental health services for vulnerable sections of the population.

Countries also vary widely on economic and development indices such as gross domestic product (GDP) and human development indices. For example, the International Monetary Fund (IMF) ranks Qatar, an oil-rich country in the Region, number one in the world in terms of GDP per capita, while Afghanistan, which has suffered from wars and civil unrest, is ranked number 171 (10). Consequently, Qatar's governmental expenditure on health per capita in 2007 was US$ 2607, while that of Afghanistan in the same year was only US$ 10 per capita. Seven countries in the Region are in complex emergency situations, namely, Iraq, Afghanistan, Pakistan, occupied Palestinian territory, Somalia, Sudan and Yemen.

1.3 Atlas projects

The WHO mental health and substance abuse programme has published a series of Atlas projects, including the Atlas of child and adolescent mental health resources (11), which was published in 2005 (Annex 2). The child and adolescent mental health atlas was a collaborative initiative between WHO, the World Psychiatric Association and the International Association of Child and Adolescent Psychiatry and Allied Professions. The Atlas provided a global overview of policies, programmes, services and resources for child and adolescent mental health. Participation of countries from the Region was, however, low as only eight countries participated (38.5%).

This Atlas is modelled after the 2005 Atlas project. However, the questionnaire was modified to collect information relevant to the Region with its unique demographic, cultural, religious and social attributes and was only administered in the Region. An attempt was made to include all countries but it was only possible to collect data from 19 countries (86.3%). Data could not be collected from Jordan, Lebanon or Qatar. Participating countries are listed according to World Bank income categories (Table 1).

1.4 Objectives of the Atlas

The overall aim of the Atlas is to increase the knowledge and understanding of the legal and policy frameworks, available resources and sociocultural factors impacting on the organization of child, adolescent and maternal mental health systems in the Region. The findings should be disseminated to policy-makers, health professionals, sister United Nations agencies and nongovernmental organizations and used for planning services and interventions for child, adolescent and maternal mental health at regional and country levels.

Table 1. Countries participating in the Atlas project according to income category	
Income category (gross national income per capita)	Country
Low-income economies (US$ 995 or less)	Afghanistan
	Somalia
Lower-middle-income economies (US$ 996 to US$ 3945)	Djibouti
	Egypt
	Iraq
	Morocco
	Pakistan
	Occupied Palestinian territory
	Sudan
	Syrian Arab Republic
	Tunisia
	Yemen
Upper-middle-income economies (US$ 3946 to US$ 12 195)	Islamic Republic of Iran
	Libyan Arab Jamahiriya
High-income economies (US$ 12 196 or more)	Bahrain
	Kuwait
	Oman
	Saudi Arabia
	United Arab Emirates

The data collected on child, adolescent and maternal mental health included information on:

- policies and legislation
- surveillance systems
- service delivery systems
- human resources
- sources of financing
- availability of psychotropic medications
- social, cultural and religious factors impacting maternal, child and adolescent mental health.

1.5 Methods and limitations

The data were collected through a survey questionnaire based on a modified version of the WHO Atlas for child and adolescent mental health resources published in 2005. Some of the questions were modified for clarification and new questions were added, including a section on prevention and promotion and a section on religious and cultural issues. The final questionnaire is included in Annex 2.

The questionnaire was used to collect information on the organization, delivery and utilization of child, adolescent and maternal mental health services. It consists of 10 sections – demographics, mental health policy and legislation, mental health services, mental health financing, human resources, nongovernmental organizations, data collection and quality assurance, care for special populations, medications, diagnostic testing and other treatment modalities, prevention, promotion and influence of other factors.

The questionnaire was sent to key informants from all countries of the Region. Key informants were national mental health focal points, designated by ministries of health to be responsible for mental health programmes in each country (Annex 1).

The use of key informants has limitations, including the potential lack of uniformity and reliability. This may be more evident in sections that require subjective responses (for example, the relation between religion and mental health), as opposed to sections that are data-driven (for example, health care financing and human resources). Overall, the limitations associated with using key informants were minimized by:

- selecting mental health focal points in national ministries of health as key informants – each focal point is arguably the most informed individual about resources available in their country as they oversee the national mental health programme;
- verifying information provided through face-to-face interviews with key informants;
- providing explanations of terminology and items on the questionnaire to informants on a regular basis;
- asking responders to provide reports, publications and policies, when available.

The use of a questionnaire with multiple-choice answers has inherent limitations and not all possible choices may be listed. For example, the options provided in the prevention and promotion section may not cover all measures available in different countries. There was an attempt to minimize this limitation by providing an "Other" option that allowed for free text entries.

This report presents some of the most significant findings from the data collected.

2. Public policy and legislation

2.1 Child and adolescent mental health

Child and adolescent mental health is addressed in some form in national policies of the majority of countries in the Region (Figure 1). In 16% of the 19 surveyed countries national child and adolescent mental health policies do not exist.

Official legislation that acknowledges the rights of children and adolescents (in addition to the UN Convention on the Rights of the Child) is present in 17 out of the 19 countries surveyed (Figure 2). Laws specifically striving to protect children and adolescents in terms of abuse, confidentiality and informed consent are present in the majority of countries surveyed.

Although 10 countries in the Region have a child and adolescent mental health programme (Bahrain, Djibouti, Egypt, Islamic Republic of Iran, Kuwait, Oman, Saudi Arabia, Somalia, United Arab Emirates and Yemen), 6 do not. One country has guidelines regarding access to care only, while another only includes a public education (awareness-raising) component (Figure 3).

2.2 Maternal mental health

Maternal mental health is identified as a priority in national policies of 10 countries in the Region (Djibouti, Islamic Republic of Iran, Libyan Arab Jamahiriya, Oman, Pakistan, occupied Palestinian territory, Saudi Arabia, Somalia, Sudan and Syrian Arab Republic).

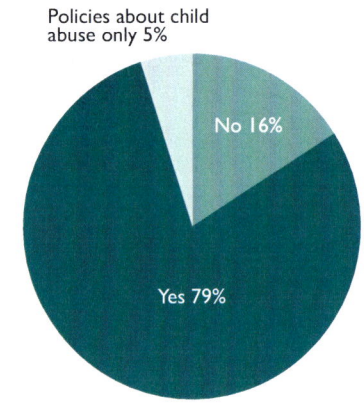

Figure 1. Percentage of countries addressing child and adolescent mental health in national policies

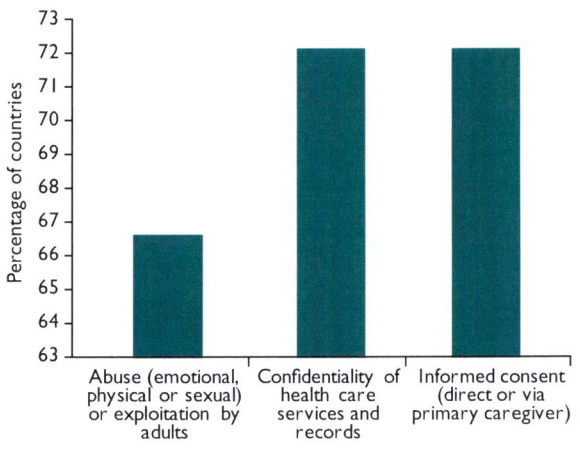

Figure 2. Percentage of countries with laws protecting children and adolescents

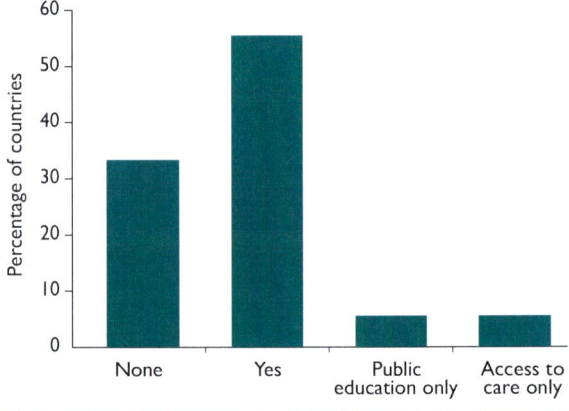

Figure 3. Existence of a child and adolescent mental health programme in countries ($n = 18$)

3. Mental health services

3.1 Child and adolescent mental health

The role of public, private and joint ventures in the provision of child and adolescent mental health services varies considerably between countries of the Region.

The public sector is the major service provider in Afghanistan, Islamic Republic of Iran, Morocco, Oman and Saudi Arabia.

The private sector is the major provider in Libyan Arab Jamahiriya, Yemen and Pakistan.

In Tunisia, the public and private sectors equally share service provision while all services in Somalia are provided by joint public–private ventures (Figure 4).

Country income category does not correlate with the role of different sectors in providing services. For example, countries where the public sector is the major provider fall into the low-income, lower-middle, upper-middle and high-income categories.

In 67% of countries surveyed child and adolescent mental health services are not provided by child and adolescent psychiatrists. The majority of service is provided by general psychiatrists, paediatricians and primary care physicians or non-physician primary health care workers (Figure 5).

In some countries, such as Afghanistan and Somalia, child and adolescent psychiatrists are not available (see Section 7).

Outpatient child and adolescent mental health care is available in most countries of the Region.

Traditional office-based care models are the most prevalent, such as outpatient departments in public hospitals and private specialists' offices.

Less traditional models of care such as mobile (outreach) services are available in very few countries (Figure 6).

67% of countries surveyed have a system for providing inpatient mental health care for mentally-ill children and adolescents (Figure 7).

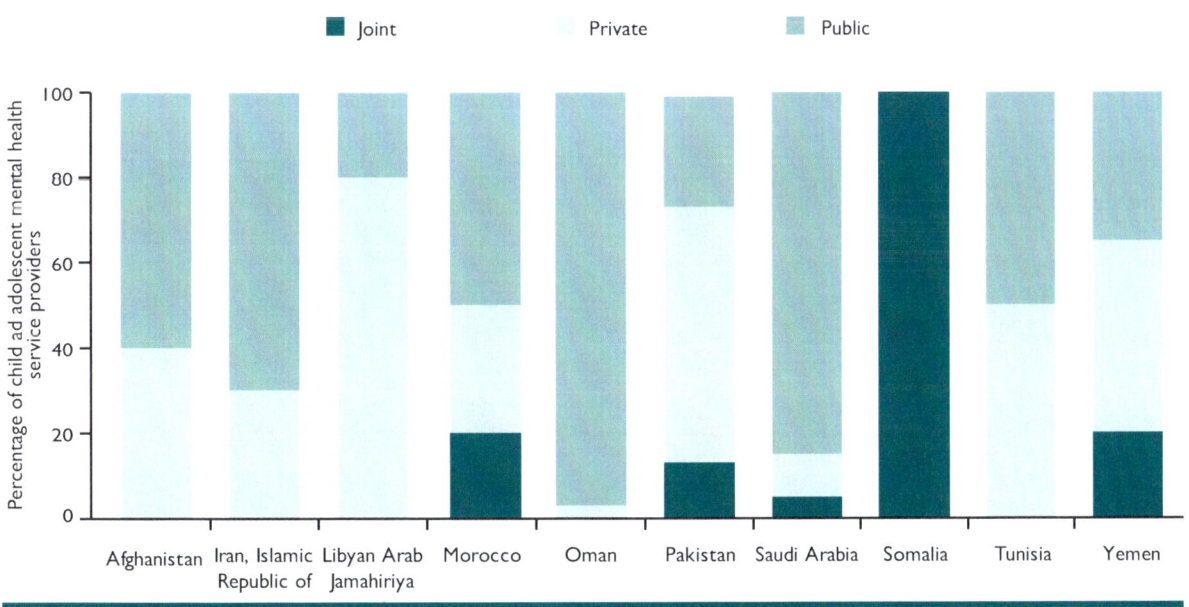

Figure 4. Distribution of child and adolescent mental health service providers, by sector

Atlas: child, adolescent and maternal mental health resources in the Eastern Mediterranean Region

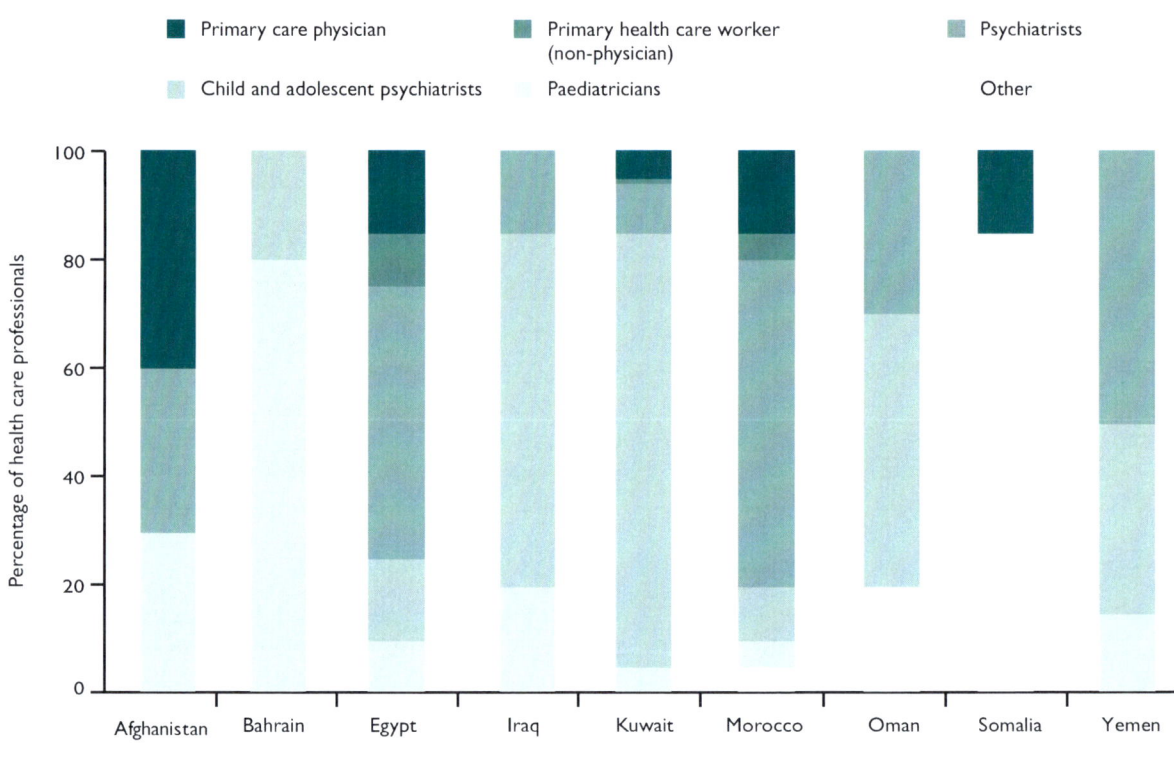

Figure 5. Distribution of health care professionals providing child and adolescent mental health services

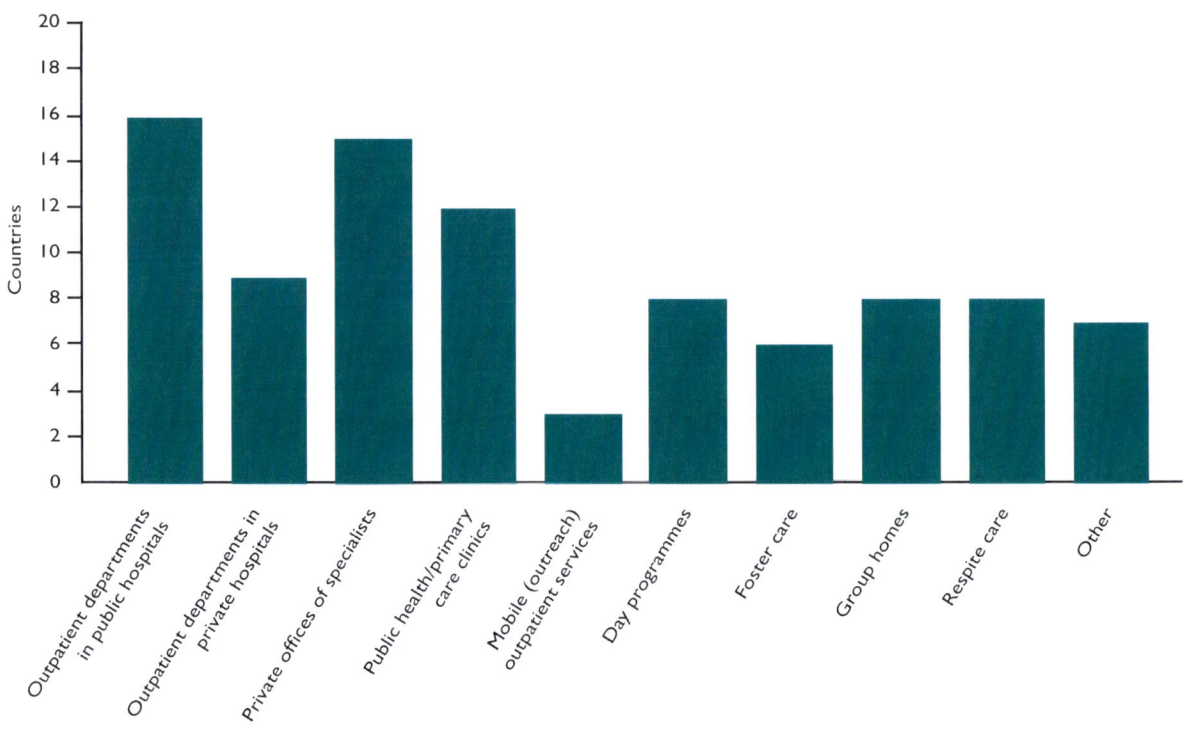

Figure 6. Types of outpatient child and adolescent mental health care in countries

Mental health services

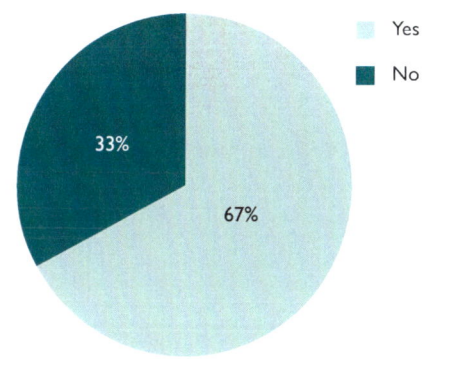

Figure 7. Percentage of countries with inpatient psychiatric facilities of any kind for mentally-ill children and adolescents (*n* = 18)

Most inpatient beds available in the Region are in psychiatric hospitals, followed by paediatric hospitals, then general hospitals and specialized psychiatric institutions (Figure 8).

A referral system exists for children and adolescents in need of mental health care in only seven of the surveyed countries. This is an alarming statistic as it means that many children in need will either not receive appropriate services or will suffer a significant delay due to the lack of defined referral channels.

The most substantial barriers to care in the Region include stigma of mental illness, lack of trained professionals and lack of mental health awareness (Figure 9).

3.2 Maternal mental health

As is the case with child and adolescent mental health, the role of the public, private, and joint ventures in the provision of maternal mental health services varies considerably between countries in the Region. The public sector is the major service provider in Islamic Republic of Iran, Morocco, Oman, Saudi Arabia and Somalia and is the sole provider in Djibouti and Kuwait. The private sector is the main maternal mental health provider in Afghanistan and Libyan Arab Jamahiriya (Figure 10).

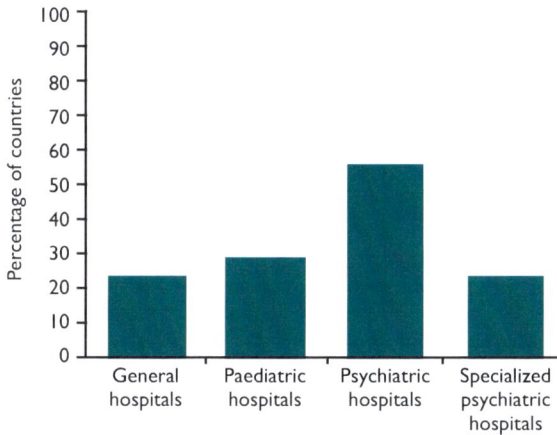

Figure 8. Types of inpatient child and adolescent mental health care

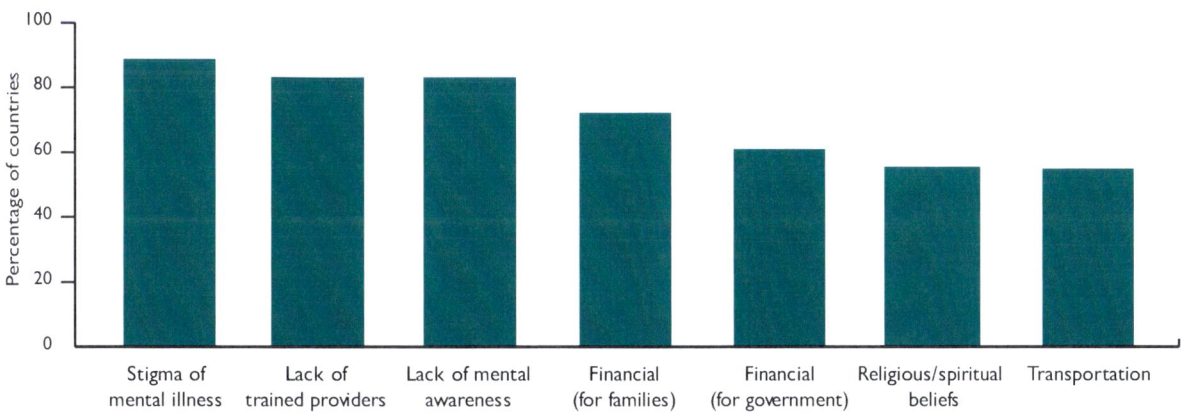

Figure 9. Barriers to child and adolescent mental health care

13

Also similar to child and adolescent mental health, country income category does not correlate with the role of different sectors in providing services. For example, countries where the public sector is the major provider fall into the low-income, lower-middle, upper-middle and high-income categories.

In 82% of countries of the Region surveyed, psychiatrists provide the majority of maternal mental health services. Somalia is an exception as the majority of maternal mental health services are provided by non-physician primary health care workers (Figure 11).

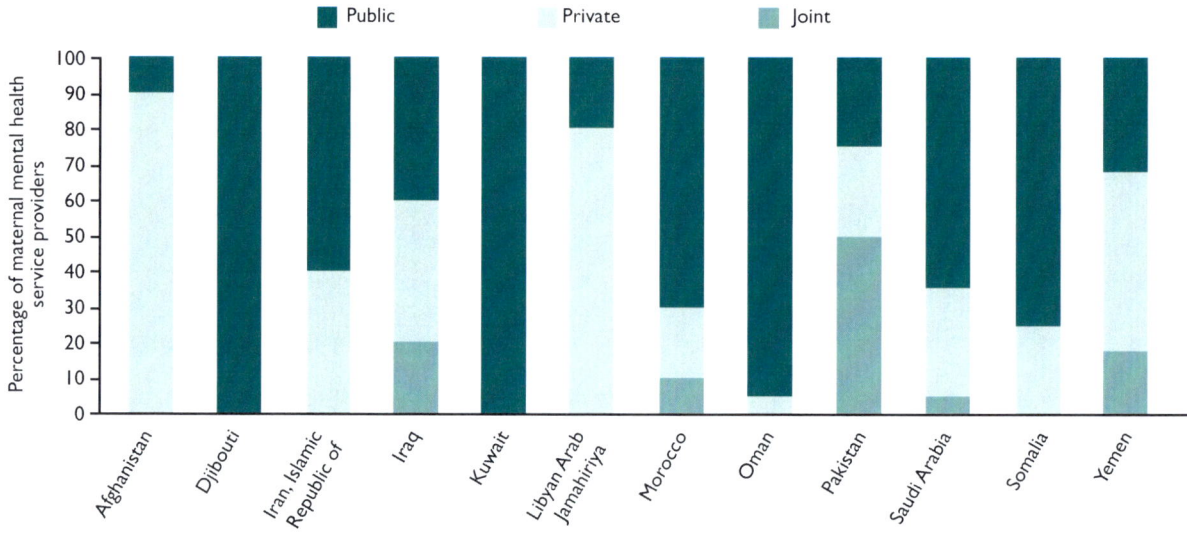

Figure 10. Maternal mental health service providers, by sector (n = 12)

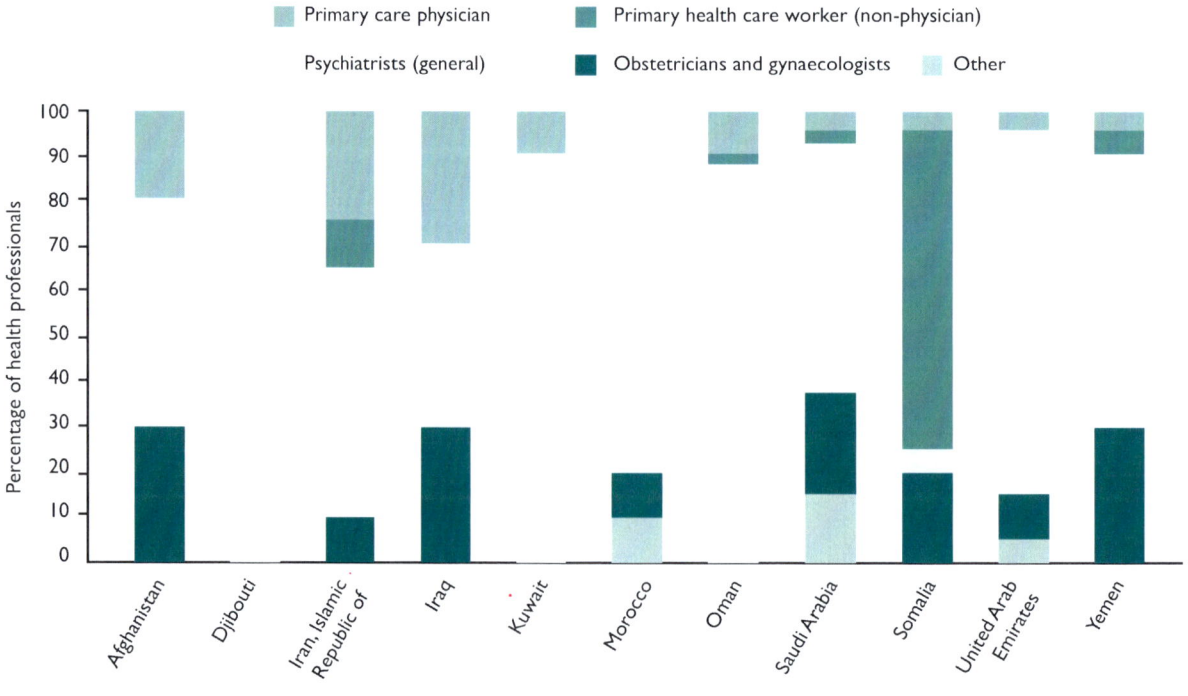

Figure 11. Distribution, by percentage, of health professionals providing maternal mental health services (n = 11)

Screening for maternal mental health problems is routinely undertaken in perinatal visits in only 3 out of the 19 surveyed countries. This poses a challenge as mental health problems in the perinatal period may go undiagnosed and thus untreated.

The most substantial barriers to maternal mental health care in the Region are the same as those impacting child and adolescent mental health, including stigma surrounding mental illness, lack of trained professionals and lack of mental health awareness (Figure 12).

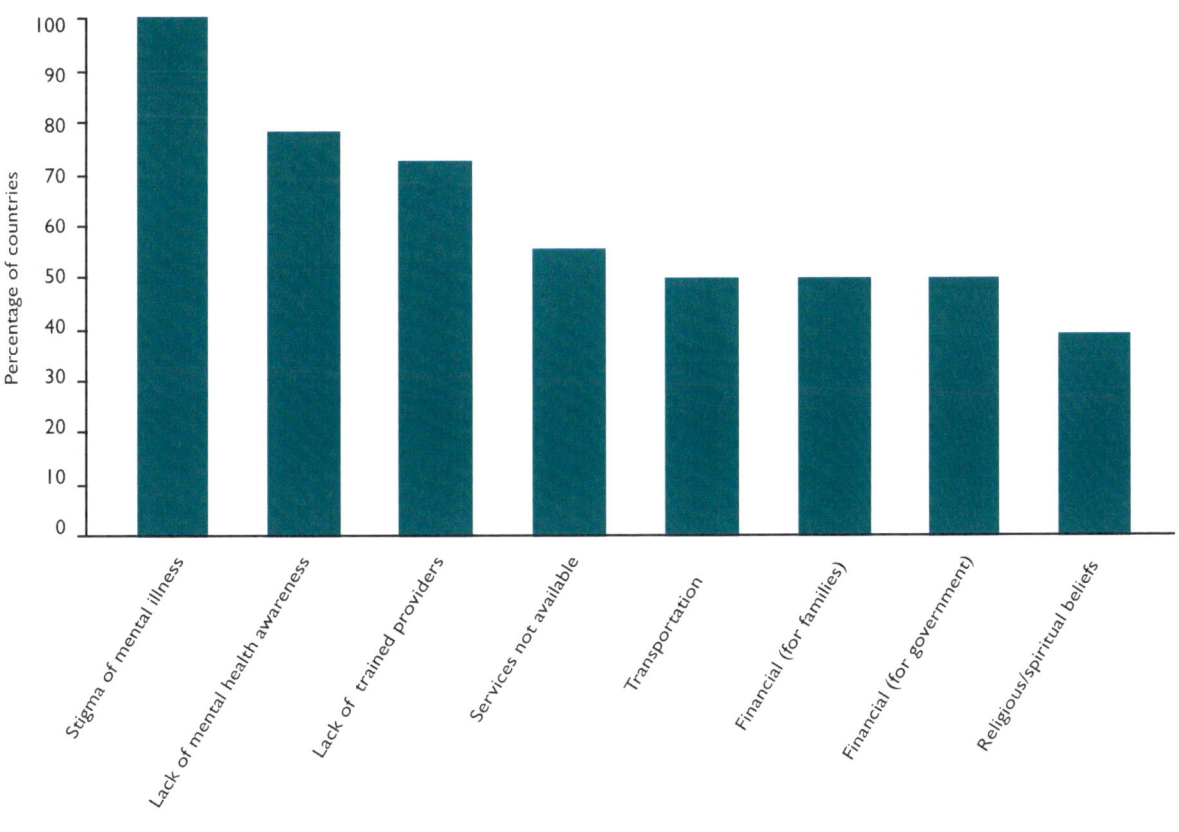

Figure 12. Barriers to maternal mental health care

4. Health care financing

The main funding source for child and adolescent mental health services in Bahrain, Djibouti, Egypt, Iraq, Kuwait, Oman, occupied Palestinian territory, Saudi Arabia and the United Arab Emirates is government funds.

Funding from individual consumers and their families (out-of-pocket) is the main source in Libyan Arab Jamahiriya, Morocco, Sudan, Syrian Arab Republic and Tunisia.

Nongovernmental organizations are the main funding source in Pakistan, Somalia and Yemen, while international grants are the main funding source in Afghanistan.

Social insurance is the main source of funding in the Islamic Republic of Iran.

Private insurance is not the main funding source in any of the countries of the Region, which is expected as penetration of private insurance in the health care market remains very low in the Region.

5. Human resources

5.1 Child and adolescent mental health

Only 4 out of 18 reporting countries have a child and adolescent psychiatry-training programme. There is a significant shortage in psychiatrists in countries. There are no practising psychiatrists in Somalia and only one psychiatrist practising in Djibouti. Among psychiatrists very few are trained/specialized in child and adolescent mental health, while among paediatricians, with the exception of one country (Yemen), no more than 1% is trained in child and adolescent mental health (Table 2).

In addition to psychiatrists and paediatricians, most countries have professionals from

Table 2. Number of psychiatrists and paediatricians trained in child and adolescent mental health in countries of the Region

Country	Number of psychiatrists	Psychiatrists specialized/ trained in child and adolescent mental health (%)	Number of paediatricians	Paediatricians trained in child and adolescent mental health (%)
Bahrain	26	15.4	62	0
Djibouti	1	0	–	0
Egypt	978	–	–	–
Iran, Islamic Republic of	1120	3	2078	0
Iraq	100	5	899	1
Kuwait	67	4.5	–	1
Libyan Arab Jamahiriya	25	10	–	–
Morocco	266	6	264	0
Oman	67	10	667	0
Pakistan	342	0.8	600	0
Occupied Palestinian territory	36	25	679	0
Saudi Arabia	501	3	1885	–
Somalia	0	–	4	0
Sudan	60	–	242	–
Syrian Arab Republic	85	31.8	–	–
Tunisia	210	–	–	–
United Arab Emirates	14	31	88	–
Yemen	25	8	250	10

other disciplines working with children and adolescents who have mental health-related problems (Figure 13).

More than two thirds of surveyed countries lack a child and adolescent mental health module in the curricula of social workers, speech therapists, primary care physicians, nurses, paediatricians, health care workers (non-physicians), occupational therapists and teachers (Figure 14).

This is a source of concern as many of these disciplines are at the forefront of both identification (teachers and primary health care workers) and treatment (paediatricians) of child and adolescent mental health problems.

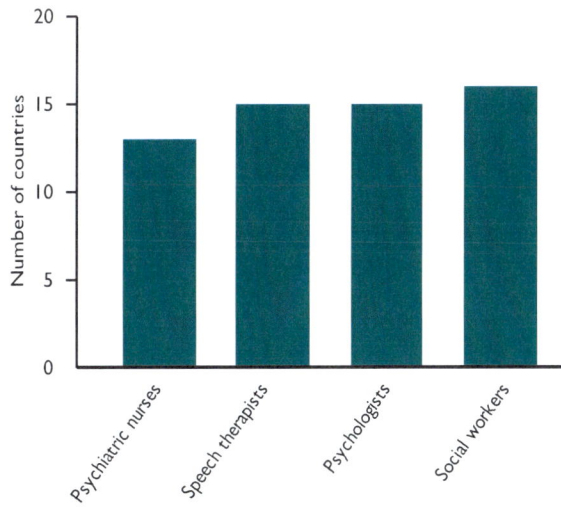

Figure 13. Other disciplines providing child and adolescent mental health care

5.2 Maternal mental health

As is the case with the educational situation in child and adolescent mental health, more than two thirds of surveyed countries lack a maternal mental health module in the curricula of obstetricians, psychologists, primary care physicians, nurses, social workers and non-physician health care workers (Figure 15). This is a source of concern as many of these disciplines are at the forefront of both identification (obstetricians) and treatment (psychologists) of maternal mental health problems.

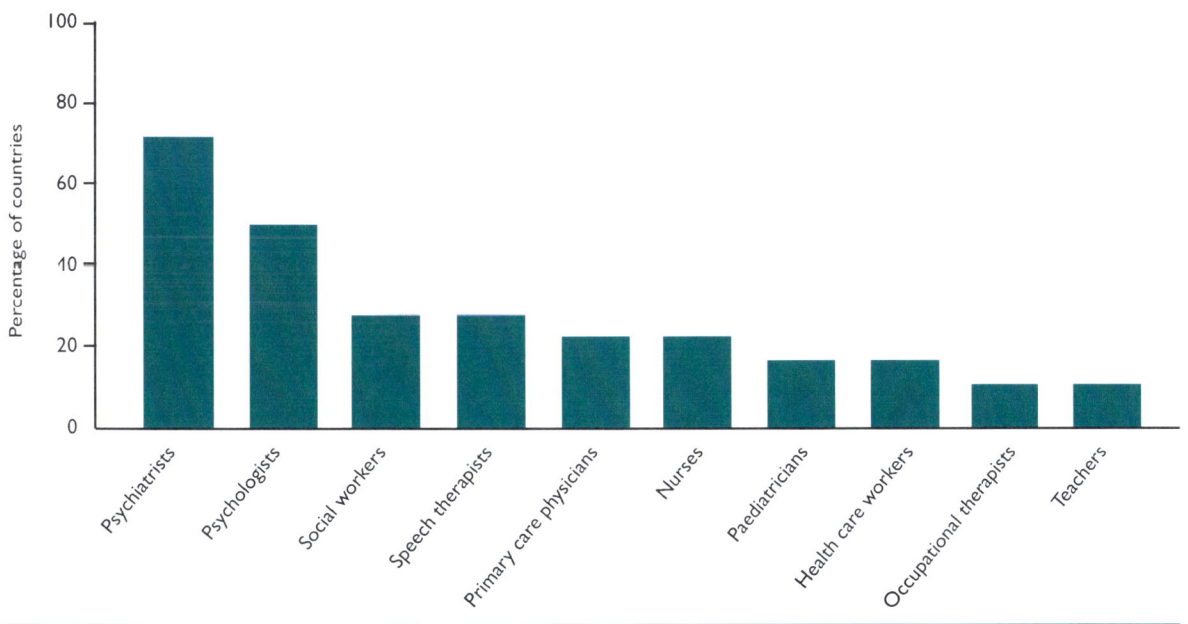

Figure 14. Percentage of countries providing training in child and adolescent mental health care within curricula

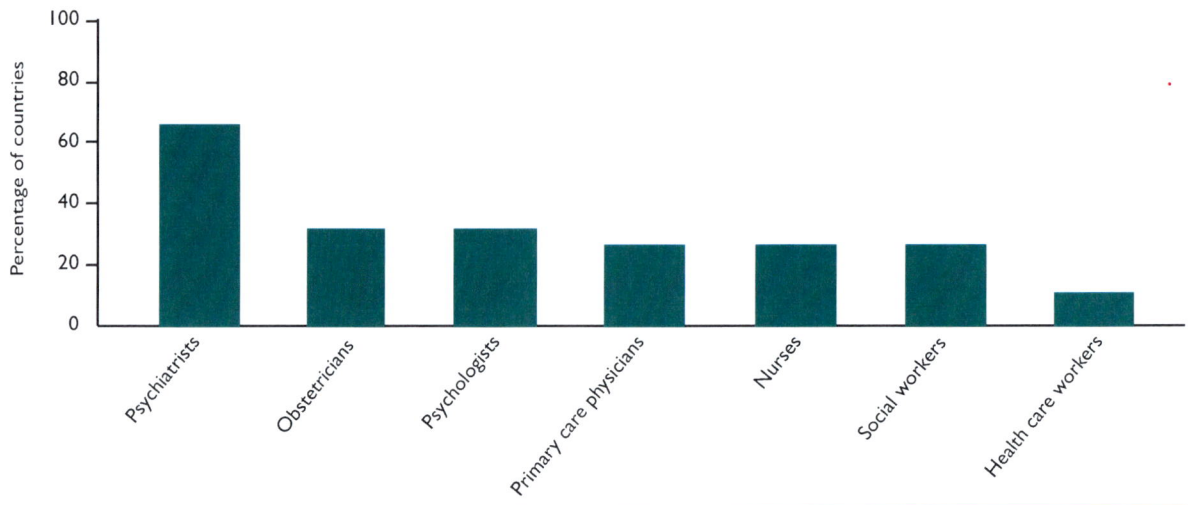

Figure 15. Percentage of countries in the Region providing training in maternal mental health care within curricula

6. Data collection and quality assurance

Only 53% of the reporting countries include information about child and adolescent mental health in their annual health reports (Figure 16), while 37% of countries include maternal mental health in annual health reports (Figure 17). Epidemiological studies on child, adolescent and maternal mental disorders in the Region are lacking and often have methodological deficiencies (Figures 18 and 19).

Few countries have data collection systems for child and adolescent suicides and for maternal suicides and infantile homicides (Figures 20 and 21), and for child and adolescent and maternal mental health services (Figures 22 and 23).

The majority of countries lack national standards of care for child and adolescent and maternal mental health (Figures 24 and 25).

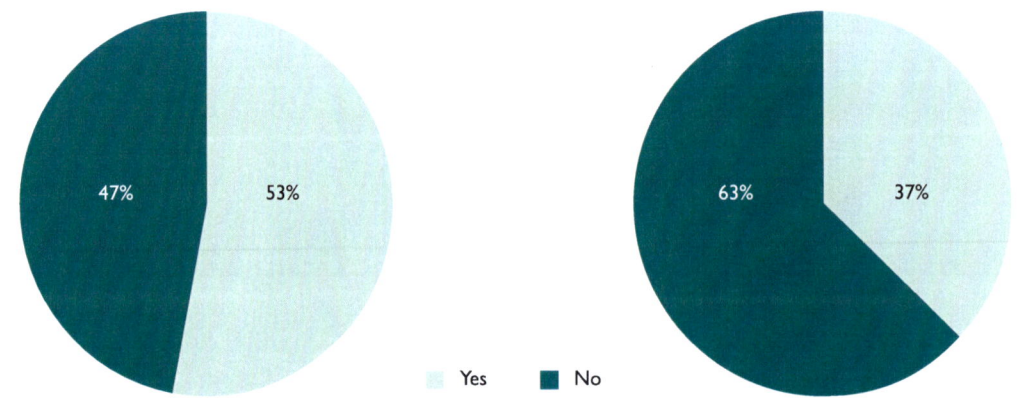

Figure 16. Percentage of countries including data on child and adolescent mental health in annual health reports

Figure 17. Percentage of countries including data on maternal mental health in annual health reports

Data collection and quality assurance

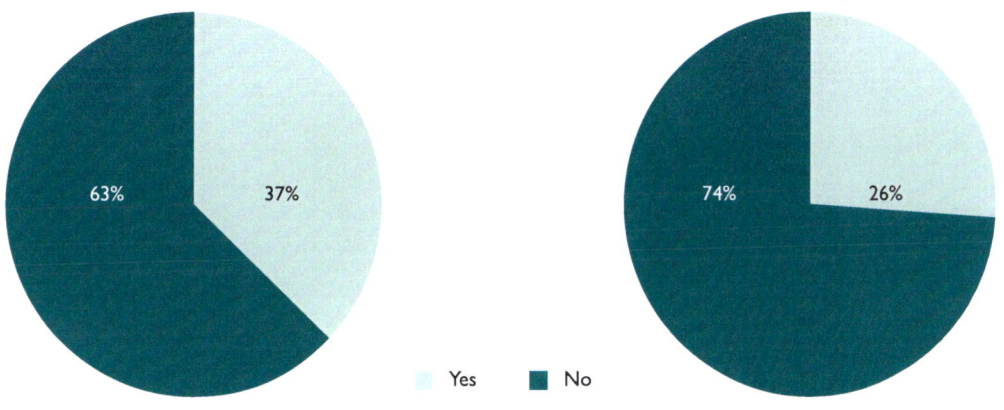

Figure 18. Percentage of countries with an epidemiological data collection system on child and adolescent mental disorders

Figure 19. Percentage of countries with an epidemiological data collection system on maternal mental disorders

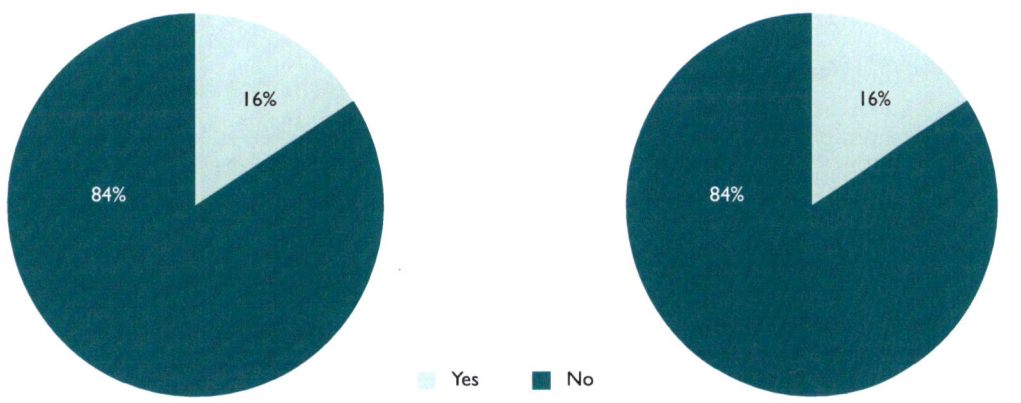

Figure 20. Percentage of countries with a surveillance system for child and adolescent suicides

Figure 21. Percentage of countries with a surveillance system for maternal suicides and infantile homicides

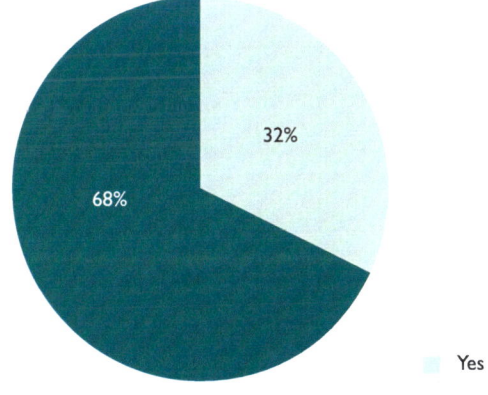 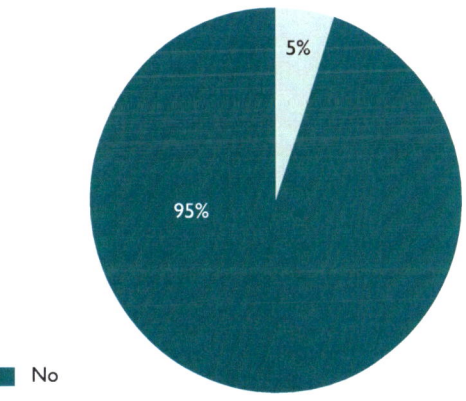

Figure 22. Percentage of countries with data collection on child and adolescent mental health services

Figure 23. Percentage of countries with data collection on maternal mental health services

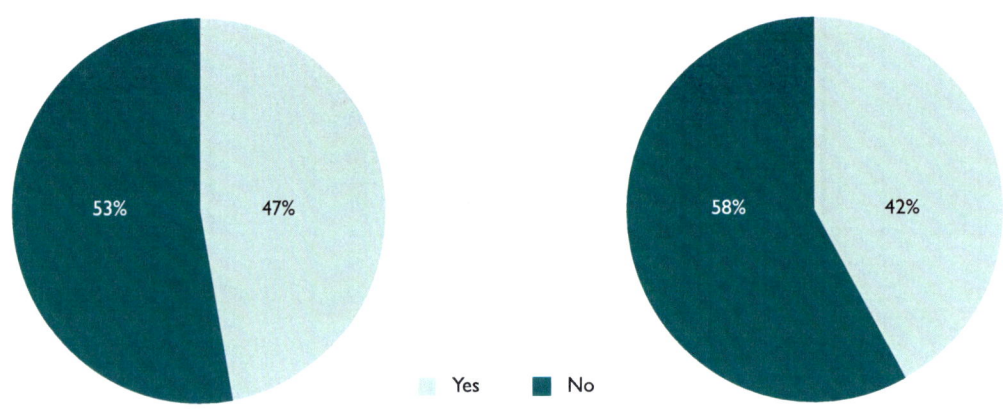

Figure 24. Percentage of countries with national standards of care for child and adolescent mental health

Figure 25. Percentage of countries with national standards of care for maternal mental health

7. Medications and other treatment modalities

Only 41% of countries surveyed include psychotropic medications for childhood mental disorders in their national list of essential medicines.

Only 39% of countries surveyed have specific provisions to control prescribing practices of medications used for children and adolescents.

In 67% of surveyed countries psychiatric medications are available for free (provided by the government sector).

Tricyclic antidepressants, anti-psychotics, anxiolytics/sedatives and anti-epileptics are available in 95% of countries in the Region. Psychostimulants, which are first-line medications for attention deficit hyperactivity disorder (ADHD), are available in primary health care in 32% of countries surveyed, while non-stimulant ADHD medications are available in 21%. Adrenergic agents, which are sometimes used as second-line ADHD agents, were available in 74% of surveyed countries. The WHO model list of essential medicines for children notes the potential importance of these medicines in children for a variety of disorders (Figure 26).

Counselling and psychotherapy are utilized routinely in almost 80% of countries in the Region. Information about access to these services and their costs is not available. Other less conventional treatments, such as naturopathic and herbal medicines, are used routinely in 16% and 26% of countries, respectively, while traditional medicines are routinely used in half of the countries (Figure 27).

Medications and other treatment modalities

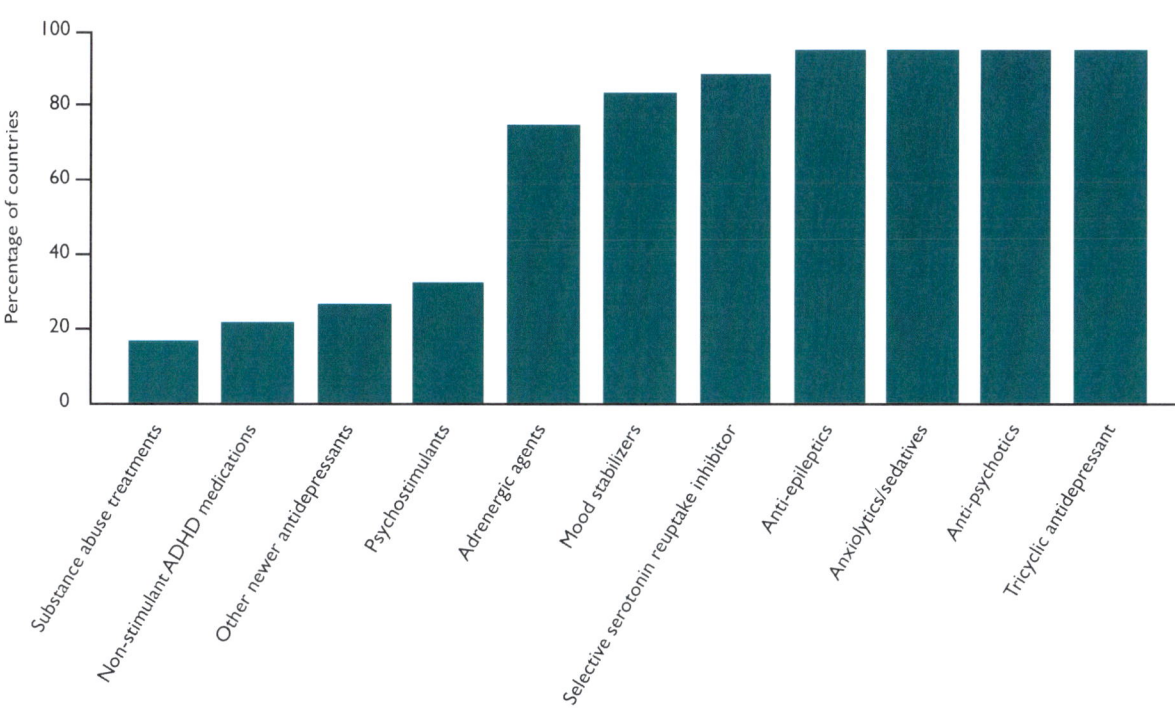

Figure 26. Percentage of countries with different categories of psychotropic medicines available in primary health care

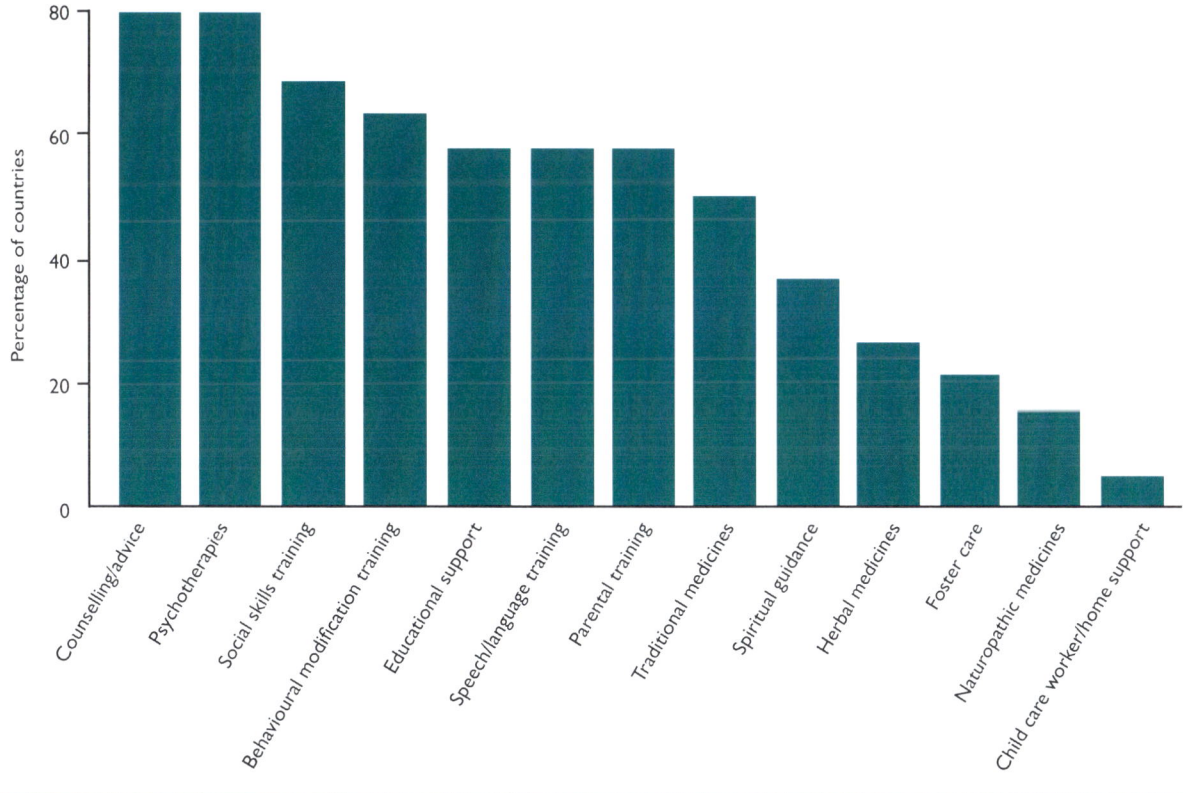

Figure 27. Percentage of countries routinely using other treatments in child and adolescent mental health

8. Child and adolescent mental health promotion and prevention of psychiatric problems

Nutritional supplementation programmes, which have a significant impact on promoting both physical and mental health, are implemented in 72% of countries in the Region.

Programmes that are specific to mental health promotion and the prevention of psychiatric morbidity, such as peer support groups, are available in 22% of countries surveyed, suicide prevention hotlines in 17% and early child stimulation in 11% (Figure 28).

School counselling services are available in 61% of surveyed countries, and are being piloted in another 6% of countries (Figure 29).

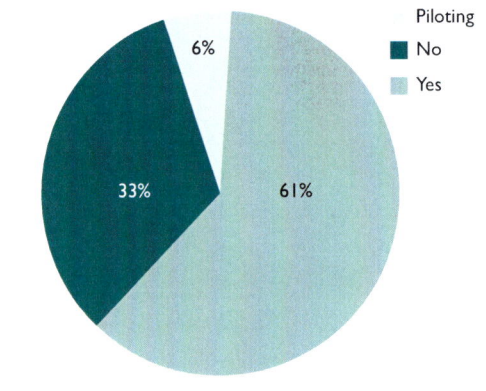

Figure 29. Percentage of countries providing school counselling services

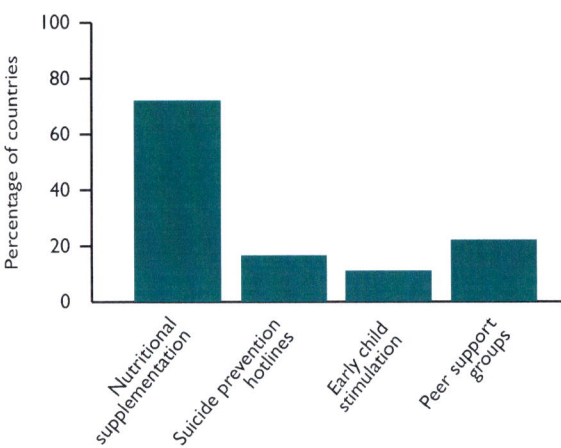

Figure 28. Percentage of countries implementing child and adolescent mental health prevention and promotion programmes

9. Religion and mental health

In two thirds of countries there is a perception that religion encourages the seeking of mental health care or is neutral in that regard, while in one third of countries it is perceived as "interfering" with the seeking of mental health care.

In the majority of countries (56.25%) religious leaders (imams, priests) are perceived as having little awareness regarding mental health issues, while in 37.5% of countries they are perceived as having some level of awareness, and in 6.25% as having a high level of awareness.

Religious beliefs are perceived to play a role in the prevention of suicides and substance abuse disorders in 94.1% of countries. Religious beliefs are perceived to play a role in the prevention of anxiety disorders in 66.7% of countries, mood disorders in 46.7%, and psychotic disorders in 28.6% (Figure 30).

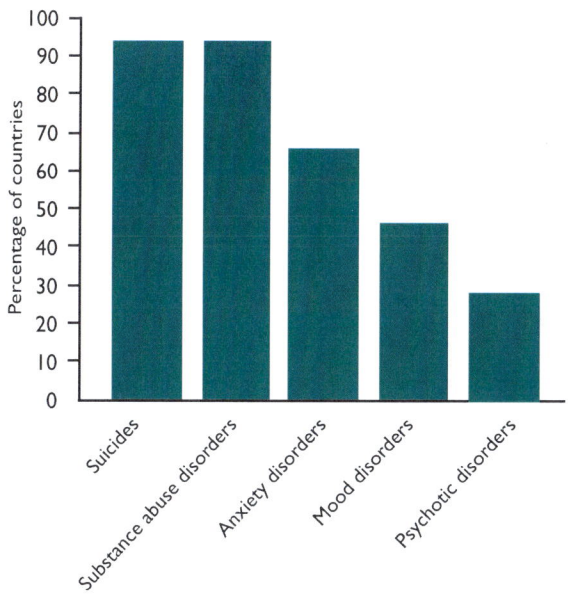

Figure 30. The role of religious beliefs in preventing mental health disorders

10. Key findings

- National policies and official legislation addressing child and adolescent mental health are present in the majority of countries in the Region. However, only 56% of countries in the Region have a child and adolescent mental health programme that would allow these policies to be implemented. It is unknown whether specified funds are allocated for such implementation.
- The roles of the public, private and joint ventures in the provision of child, adolescent and maternal mental health services varies considerably between countries in the Region.
- Referral systems for those in need of child and adolescent mental health services are available only in a few countries in the Region.
- The most substantial barriers to care for both child, adolescent and maternal mental health include stigma surrounding mental illness, lack of trained professionals and lack of mental health awareness.
- In only 3 out of the 19 surveyed countries is screening for maternal mental health problems routinely undertaken in perinatal visits.
- There is a significant shortage of human capital in child and adolescent mental health in the Region, including psychiatrists and particularly those qualified in child and adolescent mental health. In some countries, such as Afghanistan and Somalia, child and adolescent psychiatrists are non-existent.
- More than two thirds of surveyed countries lack a child and adolescent mental health module in the curricula of social workers, speech therapists, primary care physicians, nurses, paediatricians, health care workers (non-physicians), occupational therapists and teachers. This is a cause for concern as these professionals are at the forefront of identifying and providing services for children and adolescents with mental health disorders in countries of the Region.
- Training programmes in child and adolescent psychiatry are available in only 4 countries of the Region.
- More than two thirds of surveyed countries also lack a maternal mental health module in the curricula of obstetricians, psychologists, primary care physicians, nurses, social workers and health care workers (non-physicians). Again, this is a cause for concern as these professionals are at the forefront of identifying and providing maternal mental health services in countries.
- There are substantial deficits in data collection systems in child, adolescent and maternal mental health, including data on suicide rates, health services, etc., as well as epidemiological studies.

- The majority of countries lack national standards of care for child and adolescent mental health and maternal mental health.
- Only 41% of countries in the Region include psychotropic medications for childhood mental disorders in their national list of essential medicines, and only 39% have specific provisions to control prescribing practices for these medications.
- In 67% of surveyed countries psychiatric medications are available for free (provided by the governmental sector).
- Tricyclic antidepressants, anti-psychotics, anxiolytics/sedatives and anti-epileptics are available in 95% of countries in the Region. Psychostimulants, which are first-line medications for ADHD, are available in primary health care in 32% of countries surveyed while non-stimulant ADHD medications are available in 21%.
- Counselling and psychotherapy are used routinely in almost 80% of countries in the Region, and traditional medicines in half of the countries, while other less conventional treatments, such as naturopathic and herbal medicines, are routinely used in only a few countries.
- The availability and coverage of programmes for mental health promotion and the prevention of psychiatric morbidity, such as peer support groups, suicide prevention hotlines and child stimulation programmes, is limited.
- While in most countries religion is perceived to play a preventive role in psychiatric disorders and to not interfere in seeking mental health care, religious leaders are perceived as having little awareness regarding mental health issues.

References

1. Done DJ et al. Childhood antecedents of schizophrenia and affective illness: social adjustment at ages 7 and 11. *British Medical Journal (Clinical Research Ed.)*, 1994, 309:699–703.

2. Rutter M. Psychopathology and development. In: Childhood antecedents of adult psychiatric disorder. *The Australian and New Zealand Journal of Psychiatry*, 1984, 18:225–234.

3. Merikangas KR, Nakamura EF, Kessler RC. Epidemiology of mental disorders in children and adolescents. *Dialogues in Clinical Neuroscience*, 2009, 11:7–20.

4. Shatkin JP, Belfer ML. The global absence of child and adolescent mental health policy. *Child and Adolescent Mental Health*, 2004, 9:104–108.

5. Remschmidt H, Belfer ML. Mental health care for children and adolescents worldwide: a review. *World Psychiatry; Official Journal of the World Psychiatric Association (WPA)*, 2005, 4:147–153.

6. Hamoda HM, Belfer M. Challenges in international collaboration in child and adolescent psychiatry. *Journal of Child and Adolescent Mental Health*, 2010, 2(22):83–89.

7. World Health Organization.(http://www.who.int/mental_health/prevention/suicide/MaternalMH/en/index.html, accessed 20 October 2010).

8. Mann R, Gilbody S, Adamson J. Prevalence and incidence of postnatal depression: what can systematic reviews tell us? *Archives of Women's Mental Health*, 2010, 13:295–305.

9. *Demographic, social and health indicators for countries of the Eastern Mediterranean, 2010.* Cairo, Regional Office for the Eastern Mediterranean, 2010.

10. International Monetary Fund. World Economic Outlook database, October 2009 (http://www.imf.org/external/pubs/ft/weo/2009/02/weodata/index.aspx, accessed 24 June 2011).

11. *Atlas: child and adolescent mental health resources. Global concerns: implications for the future.* Geneva, Switzerland, World Health Organization, 2005 (http://www.who.int/mental_health/resources/Child_ado_atlas.pdf, accessed 24 June 2011).

Annex 1

List of respondents

Country	Respondents	Position
Afghanistan	Dr Alia Ibrahimzai	Director, Mental Health and Drug Demand Reduction, Ministry of Public Health
Bahrain	Dr Sharifa Bucheeri	Consultant Family Physician, National Mental Health Focal Point
Djibouti	Dr Idd Waîs Ibrahim	National Mental Health Focal Point
Egypt	Fahmy Bahgat	Head of Planning, Monitoring and Evaluation Directorate, General Secretariat for Mental Health, Ministry of Health
Islamic Republic of Iran	Dr Ahmad Hajebi	Director of Mental Health Department, Ministry of Health
Iraq	Dr Emad A. Abdulghani	National Adviser for Mental Health, Ministry of Health
Kuwait	Dr Haya Al-mutairi	Focal Point for Mental Health, Ministry of Health
Libyan Arab Jamahirya	Dr Ali M. Elroey	Professor of Psychiatry, Benghazi Psychiatry Hospital
Morocco	Dr Fadoua Rahhaoui	Specialist in Public Health, Ministry of Public Health
Oman	Dr Mahmoud Z. Al-Abri	Executive Director, Ibn-Sena Psychiatric Hospital and National Focal Point for Substance Abuse
Pakistan	Dr Fareed A Minhas	Head, Institute Of Psychiatry, Director, WHO Collaborating Centre, Benazir Bhutto Hospital
Occupied Palestinian territory	Dr Hazem Ashour	President of Mental Health Unit, Ministry of Health, Jerusalem, occupied Palestinian territory
Saudi Arabia	Dr Abdulhameed A. Al-Habeeb	Director General of Mental Health and Social Services, Ministry of Health
Somalia	Abdirahman A. Awale	National focal point Mental Health and Substance abuse Ministry of Health
Sudan	Zeinat B. Sanhori	National Mental Health Coordinator, Federal Ministry of Health
Syrian Arab Republic	Eyad Yanes	Head of Mental Health Department, Ministry of Health
Tunisia	Dr Samira Milad	Director of Mental Health, Ministry of Public Health
United Arab Emirates	Saleha K. Bin Thiban	Director of Al Amal Hospital, and National Mental Health Focal Point, Federal Ministry of Health, United Arab Emirates, Dubai
Yemen	Mohamed A. Al-Khulaidi	Director, Mental Health National Programme

Annex 2

Questionnaire

Country resources for child, adolescent and maternal mental health in the Region

Name of country: _____

Date of completion: Month [   ]   Year [   ]

Contact details of person responsible for answering questionnaire:

Name: _____

Title/position: _____

Mailing address: _____
_____

Telephone: _____   Fax: _____

E-mail: _____

When official data are unavailable, please indicate so and provide your best estimate. Please identify references and/or attach articles, when available.

1. Demographics

1.1   What is the country's total population? _____

      1.1.1 As of which year? _____

1.2   In this same year, how many people were less than 18 years old? _____

      1.2.1 What percentage of these NEEDED* mental health services? _____%

      1.2.2 What percentage of these RECEIVED mental health services? _____%

1.3   In this same year, how many females were between 15 and 49 years of age? _____

1.4   In this same year, how many females gave birth? _____

      1.4.1 What percentage of these NEEDED* mental health services after delivery? _____%

      1.4.2 What percentage of these RECEIVED mental health services? _____%

* Had a diagnosable mental illness that would benefit from treatment.

2. Mental health policy and legislation

2.1 Is child and adolescent mental health addressed in any official national policy?

☐ No - *Please go to question 2.2.*
☐ Yes* - In which type of policy is it addressed? Check all that apply.
　　☐ Health　　　☐ Human rights　　　☐ Child protection
　　☐ Mental health　☐ Social welfare　　☐ Educational policy
　　☐ Other: _____

*Please enclose a photocopy of the relevant policy section(s).

2.2 Does any official national policy acknowledge the rights of children and adolescents?

☐ No - *Please go to question 2.3.*
☐ Yes - Which rights does it acknowledge? _____
_____

2.3 Does any law specifically strive to protect children and adolescents in terms of:

2.3.1 Abuse (emotional, physical or sexual) or exploitation by adults　☐ Yes ☐ No
2.3.2 Confidentiality of health care services and records　　　　　　　☐ Yes ☐ No
2.3.3 Informed consent (direct or via primary caregiver)　　　　　　　☐ Yes ☐ No
2.3.4 Other: _____

2.4 ☐ No - *Please go to question 2.5.*
☐ Yes - In which type of legislation is it addressed? Check all that apply.
　　☐ Civil law　　　　☐ Family law
　　☐ Criminal law　　☐ Other: _____

2.5 Comments: _____
_____

2.6 Is maternal mental health identified as a priority in national policies?

☐ No - *Please go to question 2.7*
☐ Yes* - In which type of policy is it addressed? Check all that apply.
　　☐ Health (including reproductive health)　　☐ Human rights
　　☐ Mental health　　　　　　　　　　　　　　☐ Social welfare
　　☐ Labour (e.g. provisions for maternity leave, day care, and breastfeeding)
　　☐ Other: _____

2.7. Comments: _____

3. Mental health services

3.1 Does the country have a national or regional (state, provincial or district) child and adolescent mental health programme?

☐ No - *Please go to question 3.2*

☐ Yes - *What are the components of this national programme?*

3.1.1 Regulations on type of care provided	☐ Yes	☐ No
3.1.2 Regulations on competency of care providers	☐ Yes	☐ No
3.1.3 Guidelines regarding access to services	☐ Yes	☐ No
3.1.4 Public education(raising awareness of issues)	☐ Yes	☐ No

3.1.5 Other: _____

3.2 Is there a child welfare or child protection system?

☐ No - *Please go to question 3.3*

☐ Yes - Does this system have access to child and adolescent mental health services?

☐ Yes ☐ No

3.3 Is there a juvenile justice system for delinquent children and adolescents?

☐ No - *Please go to question 3.4*

☐ Yes - Does this system have access to child and adolescent mental health services?

☐ Yes ☐ No

3.4 What percentage of all child and adolescent mental health services are provided in: *(Total should equal 100%)*

3.4.1 Public sector	____%
3.4.2 Private sector	____%
3.4.3 Joint public–private sector ventures	____%

3.5 What percentage of all child and adolescent mental health services are provided solely by: *(Total should equal 100%)*

3.5.1 Primary care physicians	____%
3.5.2 Primary health care workers (non-physician)	____%
3.5.3 Psychiatrists (general)	____%
3.5.4 Psychiatrists (child and adolescent)	____%
3.5.5 Paediatricians	____%
3.5.6 Other: _____	____%

3.6 Are there specialized educational services available for children and adolescents with:

3.6.1 Behavioural problems	☐ Yes	☐ No
3.6.2 Learning disabilities	☐ Yes	☐ No
3.6.3 Speech and language delay	☐ Yes	☐ No
3.6.4 Social skills problems	☐ Yes	☐ No
3.6.5 Mental retardation	☐ Yes	☐ No
3.6.6 Other: _____	☐ Yes	☐ No

3.7 What percentage of these specialized educational services is within:
(Total should equal 100%)

    3.7.1 Public sector schools _____%
    3.7.2 Private sector schools _____%
    3.7.3 Other public sector agencies _____%
    3.7.4 Other private sector agencies _____%
    3.7.5 Other locations:_____%

3.8 Is there a system of providing community-based outpatient care (includes those provided by primary health care, paediatrics or psychiatry departments in general hospitals) for mentally-ill children and adolescents?

    3.8.1 Outpatient departments in public hospitals   ☐ Yes* ☐ No
    3.8.2 Outpatient departments in private hospitals   ☐ Yes* ☐ No
    3.8.3 Private offices of specialists   ☐ Yes* ☐ No
    3.8.4 Public health/primary care clinics   ☐ Yes* ☐ No
    3.8.5 Mobile (outreach) outpatient services   ☐ Yes* ☐ No
    3.8.6 Day programmes   ☐ Yes* ☐ No
        *Country-wide maximum capacity:_____ children

    3.8.7 Group homes   ☐ Yes* ☐ No
        *Country-wide maximum capacity:_____ children
        Group home: residence for a special population in need of supervised living facilities.

    3.8.8 Foster care placements   ☐ Yes* ☐ No
        *Country-wide maximum capacity:_____ children
        Foster care: supervised care for delinquent or neglected children usually in an institution or substitute home.

    3.8.9 Respite care placements   ☐ Yes* ☐ No
        *Country-wide maximum capacity:_____ children
        Respite care: provision of short-term, temporary relief to those caring for children who might otherwise require permanent placement in a facility outside the home.

    3.8.10 Other: _____   ☐ Yes* ☐ No
        *Country-wide maximum capacity:_____ children

3.9 Is there a system of providing inpatient mental health care for mentally-ill children and adolescents? Please indicate total number of beds countrywide.

    3.9.1 **General** hospitals (hospitals with different medical specialities)
        ☐ No
        ☐ Yes: Total beds allocated to children/adolescents: _____
            Total beds allocated to mentally-ill children/adolescents: ____

    3.9.2 **Paediatric** hospitals (hospitals for children only)
        ☐ No
        ☐ Yes: Total beds: _____
            Total number of beds allocated to mentally-ill children: _____

    3.9.3 **Psychiatric** hospitals (free-standing facilities)
        ☐ No
        ☐ Yes: Total beds allocated to children/adolescents: _____

3.9.4 Specialized inpatient psychiatric institutions for children and adolescents with mental disorders

☐ No
☐ Yes: Total number of beds: _____ Average length of stay: _____
Type: _____

3.10 Is there a designated referral system for children and adolescents with mental disorders?
☐ No ☐ Yes

3.11 If initial attempts at providing mental health care (inpatient or outpatient) are insufficient, is there access to specialist consultation? Check all that apply.

☐ No - *Please go to question 3.12*

☐ Yes, but only if family is easily able to pay for it.

☐ Yes, but only if family lives in an urban centre.

☐ Yes, with equal access regardless of financial situation.

☐ Yes, with equal access regardless of geographical location.

3.12 What is the average time from a referral to a specialist visit?

3.12.1 Referral to a general psychiatrist   months ____ days ____
3.12.2 Referral to a ghild and adolescent Psychiatrist   months ____ days ____
3.12.3 Referral to a paediatrician (for a mental health problem) months ____ days ____

3.13 What is the average travel time a referred family must endure in order to visit a specialist?
_____ hours *(or)* _____ days

3.14 Is there a publication or reference that tells about child and adolescent mental health services in your country?_____
Please give the reference and/or attach a copy of the publication(s)._____

3.15 Does the country have facilities for treatment of substance abuse (alcohol or drug) problems specifically for children and adolescents?

☐ No - *Please go to question 3.16*

☐ Yes - What are the types of services available (check all that apply)?

☐ Inpatient services   ☐ Outpatient services (individual, family or group)

☐ Residential treatment   ☐ Partial hospitalization

☐ Other_____

3.16 Does the country have facilities for mental health treatment of eating disorders (e.g. anorexia nervosa or bulimia) specifically for children and adolescents?

☐ No - *Please go to question 3.17*

☐ Yes - What are the types of services available (check all that apply)?

☐ Inpatient services   ☐ Outpatient services (individual, family or group)

☐ Residential treatment   ☐ Partial hospitalization

Other_____

3.17 Does the country have facilities for developmental problems (e.g. autism spectrum disorders) for children and adolescents?

☐ No - *Please go to question 3.18*
☐ Yes - What are the types of services available (check all that apply)?
    ☐ Inpatient services   ☐ Outpatient services (individual or group)
    ☐ Residential treatment   ☐ Partial hospitalization
    ☐ Specialized schools   ☐ Other: _____

3.18 What barriers exist to the provision of child and adolescent mental health services? Check all that apply, and circle the most significant barrier.

☐ Transportation   ☐ Financial (for government)
☐ Stigma of mental illness   ☐ Religious/spiritual beliefs
☐ Lack of trained care providers   ☐ Financial (for families)
☐ Lack of mental health awareness   ☐ Other: _____

3.19 Comments: _____

3.20 What percentage of maternal mental health services are provided in:
(Total should equal 100%)

    3.20.1 the public sector?   ____%
    3.20.2 the private sector?   ____%
    3.20.3 joint public–private sector ventures?   ____%

3.21 What percentage of all maternal mental health services are provided by:
(Total should equal 100%)

    3.21.1 Primary care physicians?   ____%
    3.21.2 Primary health care workers (non-physician)?   ____%
    3.21.3 Psychiatrists (general)?   ____%
    3.21.4 Obstetricians and gynaecologists?   ____%
    3.21.5 Other? _____   ____%

3.22 Are there other specialized services available for mothers in the perinatal period?

    3.22.1 Visiting nurses   ☐ Yes ☐ No
    3.22.2 Support groups   ☐ Yes ☐ No
    3.22.3 Hotlines   ☐ Yes ☐ No
    3.22.4 Other: _____   ☐ Yes ☐ No

3.23 Is there a system of providing community-based outpatient care for mothers with mental illness in the postpartum period?

    3.23.1 Outpatient departments in public hospitals   ☐ Yes ☐ No
    3.23.2 Outpatient departments in private hospitals   ☐ Yes ☐ No
    3.23.3 Private offices of specialists   ☐ Yes ☐ No
    3.23.4 Public health/primary care clinics   ☐ Yes ☐ No

	3.23.5 Mobile (outreach) outpatient services	☐ Yes ☐ No
	3.23.6 Day patient programmes	☐ Yes ☐ No
	3.23.7 Other: _____	☐ Yes ☐ No

3.24 What barriers exist to the provision of maternal mental health services? Check all that apply, and circle the most significant barrier.

☐ Services not available   ☐ Transportation   ☐ Financial (or government)
☐ Financial (for families)   ☐ Stigma of mental illness   ☐ Religious/spiritual beliefs
☐ Lack of trained treatment providers
☐ Lack of mental health awareness
☐ Other_____

3.25 Is screening for maternal mental health problems routinely undertaken in perinatal visits?

☐ Yes   ☐ No_____

3.26 Is there a publication or reference that tells about maternal mental health services n your country?_____
Please give the reference and/or attach a copy of the publication(s)._____

3.27 Comments: _____
_____

4. Child, adolescent, maternal mental health financing

4.1 How are child and adolescent mental health services mainly funded? Choose only one of:

☐ Consumer/patient/family ☐ Private insurance
☐ Tax-based government funding ☐ Social insurance
☐ International grants
☐ Other:_____
☐ Nongovernmental organization: _____

4.2 What percentage of total child and adolescent mental health funding does this primary source of funding represent?

☐ 100% ☐ 66% ☐ 33% ☐ 0%
☐ 75%   ☐ 50% ☐ 25% ☐ Other: _____ %

4.3 Are there other sources of funding for child and adolescent mental health services?

☐ No *Please go to question 4.4*
☐ Yes - Please **list** the top three other sources:*

1. _____ _____ %
2. _____ _____ %
3. _____ _____ %

* *Please note total % adding 4.2 and 4.3 should not exceed 100%.*

4.4 What role, if any, does the source of funding play in determining which child and adolescent mental health services are provided?
_____
_____

4.5 What subsidized or free government benefits are provided to a family who has a child or adolescent with a mental illness? Please indicate amounts (in local currency), where applicable.

☐ No benefits are provided - *Please go to question 4.6*
☐ Disability pension (_____/ month) ☐ Institutional care
☐ Specialized education programmes   ☐ Parental training or education
☐ Respite/practical help for caregiver ☐ Stipend (_____/ month)
☐ Medical (including psychiatric care   ☐ Other: _____

4.6 Comments:_____
_____

4.7 How are maternal mental health services *mainly* funded? Choose only **one** of:

☐ Consumer/patient/family   ☐ Private insurance
☐ Tax-based government funding   ☐ Social insurance
☐ International grants   ☐ Other:_____
☐ Nongovernmental organization: _____

4.8 What percentage of maternal mental health funding does this primary source of funding represent?

☐ 100% ☐ 66% ☐ 33% ☐ 0%
☐ 75%   ☐ 50% ☐ 25% ☐ Other: _____ %

4.9 Are there other sources of funding maternal mental health services?

☐ No *Please go to question 4.10.*
☐ Yes- Please **list** the top three other sources:*
1. _____ _____%
2. _____ _____%
3. _____ _____%

* *Please note total % adding 4.8 and 4.9 should not exceed 100%.*

4.10 What role, if any, does the source of funding play in determining which maternal mental health services are provided?
_____
_____

4.11 Comments: _____
_____

5. Human resources

5.1 How many *psychiatrists* are practising in the country? _____

    5.1.1 What percentage of these psychiatrists has received specialized training in child and adolescent psychiatry? _____ %

    5.1.2 Do you have an in-country child and adolescent psychiatry training programme?
    ☐ Yes   ☐ No   How many? _____

    5.1.3 What is the duration of the training programme? _____

    5.1.4 Does the programme lead to a certificate of specialization?
    ☐ Yes   No

    5.1.5 What percentage of trained child and adolescent psychiatrists receive their training outside your country? _____ %

    5.1.6 For those who are trained outside the country, who mainly sponsors their training?

    ☐ They are self-sponsored (includes family support)

    ☐ The government through ministry of health or public university hospitals

    ☐ Scholarships through the host country

    ☐ Private companies, foundations or donors

    ☐ Other: _____

5.2 How many practising paediatricians exist in your country? _____

    5.2.1 How many *paediatricians* see children and adolescents who have mental health-related problems? _____

    5.2.2 What percentage of paediatricians in your country have received specialized training in child and adolescent psychiatry? _____ %

5.3 Which other professionals work with children and adolescents who have mental health-related problems?
Please check all that apply, and estimate the percentage for each profession.

5.3.1 Psychiatric nurses	☐ Yes ____%	☐ No
5.3.2 Psychologists	☐ Yes ____%	☐ No
5.3.3 Social workers	☐ Yes ____%	☐ No
5.3.4 Speech and language therapists	☐ Yes ____%	☐ No
5.3.5 Other: _____	☐ Yes ____%	☐ No

5.4 Is there a child and adolescent mental health training module incorporated into the education of all in-country trained?

5.4.1 Psychiatrists	☐ Yes	☐ No	☐ None trained
5.4.2 Paediatricians	☐ Yes	☐ No	☐ None trained
5.4.3 Primary care physicians	☐ Yes	☐ No	☐ None trained
5.4.4 Nurses	☐ Yes	☐ No	☐ None trained
5.4.5 Health care workers	☐ Yes	☐ No	☐ None trained
5.4.6 Psychologists	☐ Yes	☐ No	☐ None trained
5.4.7 Social workers	☐ Yes	☐ No	☐ None trained

	5.4.8 Speech and language therapists	☐ Yes	☐ No	☐ None trained
	5.4.9 Occupational therapists	☐ Yes	☐ No	☐ None trained
	5.4.10 Teachers	☐ Yes	☐ No	☐ None trained
	5.4.11 Other: _____	☐ Yes	☐ No	☐ None trained

5.5 Comments: _____

5.6 What percentage of obstetricians has received training in maternal mental health? _____ %

5.7 Is there a maternal mental health training module incorporated into the education of all in-country trained?

5.7.1 Psychiatrists	☐ Yes	☐ No	☐ None trained
5.7.2 Obstetricians	☐ Yes	☐ No	☐ None trained
5.7.3 Primary care physicians	☐ Yes	☐ No	☐ None trained
5.7.4 Nurses	☐ Yes	☐ No	☐ None trained
5.7.5 Health care workers	☐ Yes	☐ No	☐ None trained
5.7.6 Psychologists	☐ Yes	☐ No	☐ None trained
5.7.7 Social workers	☐ Yes	☐ No	☐ None trained
5.7.8 Other: _____	☐ Yes	☐ No	☐ None trained

6. Nongovernmental organizations

6.1 With which child and adolescent mental health activities have nongovernmental organizations (NGOs) been involved? *Check all that apply.*

☐ None - *Please go to question 6.8.*
☐ Advocacy
☐ Promotion
☐ Policy and systems development
☐ Training
☐ Treatment/"Field work"
☐ Rehabilitation
☐ Prevention
☐ Other: _____

6.2 Please list two of these NGOs.

NGO 1: _____ NGO 2: _____

6.3 Have NGOs collaborated with your country regarding their child and adolescent mental health programme development?

☐ Yes ☐ Partially ☐ No

6.4 Have NGOs linked their efforts with existing child and adolescent mental health services?

☐ Yes ☐ Partially ☐ No

6.5 Have NGOs ensured programme maintenance/continuity even after they withdraw from your country?

☐ Yes ☐ Partially ☐ No

6.6 Are NGO-sponsored child and adolescent mental health programmes accepted by the communities they were meant to serve?

☐ Yes ☐ Some programmes ☐ Some communities ☐ No

6.7 Comments: _____

6.8 With which maternal mental health activities have NGOs been involved? Check all that apply.

☐ None - *Please go to question 7.*
☐ Advocacy
☐ Promotion
☐ Policy and systems development
☐ Training
☐ Treatment/"Field Work"
☐ Rehabilitation
☐ Prevention
☐ Other: _____

6.9 Please list two of these NGOs.

NGO 1: _____ NGO 2: _____

6.10 Have NGOs collaborated with your country regarding maternal mental health?

☐ Yes ☐ Partially ☐ No

6.11 Have NGOs linked their efforts with existing maternal mental health services?

☐ Yes ☐ Partially ☐ No

6.12 Have NGOs ensured programme maintenance/continuity even after they withdraw from your country?

☐ Yes ☐ Partially ☐ No

6.13 Are NGO-sponsored maternal mental health programmes accepted by the communities they were meant to serve?

☐ Yes ☐ Some programmes ☐ Some communities ☐ No

6.14 Comments: _____
_____

7. Data collection and quality assurance

7.1 Are child and adolescent mental health disorders included your country's annual health reporting system?

☐ Yes ☐ No

7.2 Is there any epidemiological data collection system for child and adolescent mental health disorders?

☐ Yes ☐ No

7.3 Are there any publications of epidemiological data for child and adolescent mental ☐ health disorders? ☐ Yes ☐ No

Please give the reference and/or attach a copy of the publication(s)._____

7.4 Is there any surveillance system for child and adolescent suicides in your country?

☐ Yes ☐ No

Please explain._____

What is the suicide rate for children and adolescents in your country?_____/100 000

7.5 Is there any service data collection system for child and adolescent mental health disorders?

☐ No - *Please go to question 7.6*

☐ Yes - Is there monitoring of service outcomes?
  ☐ Yes ☐ No

7.6 Are there any publications on mental health services for child and adolescent mental health disorders?

☐ Yes ☐ No

Please give the reference and/or attach a copy of the publication(s)._____

7.7 Are there national minimal standards of care expected from professionals working in child and adolescent mental health?

☐ No - *Please go to question 7.8.*

☐ Yes - How are standards maintained? Check all that apply.

☐ Professional certification and maintenance of competency

☐ In-service training

☐ Clinical supervision of workers

☐ Usage of clinical practice guidelines

☐ Other:_____

7.8 Comments:_____

7.9 Are maternal mental disorders included your country's annual health reporting system?

☐ Yes ☐ No

7.10 Is there any epidemiological data collection system for maternal mental health disorders?

☐ Yes ☐ No

7.11 Are there any publications of epidemiological data for maternal mental health disorders?

☐ Yes ☐ No

Please give the reference and/or attach a copy of the publication(s)._____

_____

7.12 Is there any surveillance system for maternal suicides or infantile homicide in your country?

☐ Yes ☐ No

Please explain._____

7.13 Is there any *service* data collection system for *maternal* mental health disorders?

☐ No - *Please go to question 7.14*

☐ Yes - Is there monitoring of service outcomes? ☐ Yes ☐ No

7.14 Are there any publications on mental health services for *maternal* mental health disorders?

☐ Yes ☐ No

Please give the reference and/or attach a copy of the publication(s).____

7.15 Are there national minimal standards of care expected from professionals working in maternal mental health?

☐ No - *Please go to question 7.16*

☐ Yes - How are standards maintained? Check all that apply.

☐ Professional certification and maintenance of competency

☐ n-service training

☐ Clinical supervision of workers

☐ Usage of clinical practice guidelines

☐ Other: _____

7.16 Comments: _____

8. Care for special populations

8.1 Which subgroups of children and adolescents have access to specially designated mental health services, tailored to the subgroup's unique needs?

- [ ] None - *Please go to question 9*
- [ ] Minority groups
- [ ] Indigenous people
- [ ] Orphans
- [ ] Runaways/ homeless
- [ ] Refugees
- [ ] Disaster-affected population
- [ ] "Seriously emotionally disturbed"
- [ ] Other: _____

8.2 Comments: _____

9. Medications, diagnostic testing and other treatment modalities

9.1 Is there a national essential medicines list of psychotropic medicines for children and adolescents?

☐ Yes ☐ No

9.2 Are there specific provisions made to control prescribing practices of medications used for children and adolescents?

☐ No - *Please go to question 9.3*

☐ Yes - What are these provisions? Check all that apply:

☐ Narcotics Control Board ☐ Level of training required

☐ Prescription auditing/reviews Other: _____

9.3 Which of the following pharmaceutical drug categories are available to the primary health care system for use in children and adolescents? Check all that apply; answer the additional questions where applicable.

☐ Psychostimulants

Are they consistently available? ☐ Yes ☐ No

Generic name of most prescribed: _____

What is it mainly used for? _____

What is the approximate cost of a 30-day supply of the least expensive medication available in this group?
US$ _____

☐ Non-stimulant ADHD medications (e.g. atomoxetine)

Are they consistently available? ☐ Yes ☐ No

Generic name of most prescribed: _____

What is the approximate cost of a 30-day supply of the least expensive medication available in this group?
US$ _____

☐ Tricyclic antidepressants

Are they consistently available? ☐ Yes ☐ No

Generic name of most prescribed: _____

What is it mainly used for? _____

What is the approximate cost of a 30-day supply of the least expensive medication available in this group?
US$ _____

☐ Selective serotonin reuptake inhibitors

Are they consistently available? ☐ Yes ☐ No

Generic name of most prescribed: _____

What is it mainly used for? _____

What is the approximate cost of a 30-day supply of the least expensive medication available in this group?
US$ _____

☐ Other newer antidepressants

    Are they consistently available?   ☐ Yes   ☐ No

    Generic name of most prescribed: _____

    What is it mainly used for? _____

What is the approximate cost of a 30-day supply of the least expensive medication available in this group?
US$ _____

☐ Anti-psychotics

    Are they consistently available?   ☐ Yes   ☐ No

    Generic name of most prescribed: _____

    What is it mainly used for? _____

What is the approximate cost of a 30-day supply of the least expensive medication available in this group?
US$ _____

☐ Mood stabilizers

    Are they consistently available?   ☐ Yes   ☐ No

    Generic name of most prescribed: _____

    What is it mainly used for? _____

What is the approximate cost of a 30-day supply of the least expensive medication available in this group?
US$ _____

☐ Anti-epileptics

    Are they consistently available?   ☐ Yes   ☐ No

    Generic name of most prescribed: _____

    What is it mainly used for? _____

What is the approximate cost of a 30-day supply of the least expensive medication available in this group?
US$ _____

☐ Anxiolytics/sedatives

    Are they consistently available?   ☐ Yes   ☐ No

    Generic name of most prescribed: _____

    What is it mainly used for? _____

What is the approximate cost of a 30-day supply of the least expensive medication available in this group?
US$ _____

Adrenergic agents (such as propranolol or clonidine)

    Are they consistently available?   Yes   No

    Generic name of most prescribed: _____

    What is it mainly used for? _____

What is the approximate cost of a 30-day supply of the least expensive medication available in this group?
US$ _____

☐ Medications for substance abuse treatment
(e.g. naltrexone, acamprosate, methadone, suboxone)

    Are they consistently available?   ☐ Yes   ☐ No

Generic name of most prescribed: _____

What is it mainly used for? _____

What is the approximate cost of a 30-day supply of the least expensive medication available in this group?
US$_____

9.4 What is the cost of psychiatric medications to the patient/family? Check all that apply.

☐ Free of cost
☐ Subsidized prices, equal amount of subsidy for all patients
☐ Subsidized prices, sliding scale of subsidy based on family finances
☐ Subsidized prices, based on other: _____
☐ Market prices

9.5 What other treatment methods are routinely used in child and adolescent mental health care? Check all that apply.

☐ Herbal medicines
☐ Naturopathic medicines
☐ Behavioural modification training
☐ Learning assistance/educational supports
☐ Childcare worker/home supports
☐ Speech/language training
☐ Psychotherapies

☐ Traditional medicines
☐ Spiritual guidance
☐ Social skills training
☐ Parental training
☐ Foster care placement
☐ Counselling/advice
☐ Other: _____

9.6 Comments: _____

10. Prevention and promotion and the influence of other factors

10.1 Which of the following programmes are available for the promotion of child and adolescent mental health and prevention of psychiatric problems? Check all that apply.

☐ Nutritional supplementation ☐ Early child stimulation
☐ Suicide prevention hotlines ☐ Peer support groups
☐ Other_____

10.2 Are counselling and mental health services provided through the school system?

☐ No - *Please go to question 10.4*
☐ Yes – Who provides these services? check all that apply
☐ Psychologists ☐ Psychiatrists
☐ Social workers ☐ Psychiatric nurses
☐ Para-professional counsellors ☐ Teachers
☐ Other_____

10.3 What proportion of primary and secondary schools have either a part-time or full-time mental health professional? _____%

10.4 What is your perception about the public's understanding of the relationship between religion and seeking mental health care?

☐ Religion interferes with seeking mental health care
☐ Neutral
☐ Religion encourages seeking mental health care

10.5 What is your perception about awareness among religious leaders (imams, priests) about mental health issues in your country?

☐ They have a high level of awareness and make referrals to mental health professionals
☐ They have some level of awareness
☐ They have little awareness
☐ They have no awareness and oppose referrals to mental health professionals

10.6. Which of the following factors is the major impediment to those seeking mental health in your country?

☐ Perception of mental illness as a weakness of faith
☐ Perception of mental illness as an act of possession by a spirit
☐ Perception of mental illness to be a result of an "evil eye"
☐ Other:_____

10.7 Do religious beliefs in your country play a role in the prevention of the following?

Suicides	☐ Yes	☐ No
Substance abuse disorders	☐ Yes	☐ No
Mood disorders	☐ Yes	☐ No
Psychotic disorders	☐ Yes	☐ No
Anxiety disorders	☐ Yes	☐ No

10.8 Please describe the positive role that social, cultural and religious factors in your country play may play in the prevention and treatment of mental illness?

1 _____
2 _____
3 _____
4 _____
5 _____

10.9 Please describe the negative role that social, cultural and religious factors in your country may play in the prevention and treatment of mental illness?

1 _____
2 _____
3 _____
4 _____
5 _____

Please return completed questionnaires, policy photocopies and articles (if indicated) at your earliest convenience to:

Thank you for your assistance.

This questionnaire is based on a modified version of the WHO Atlas project conducted in 2005.